THE
SWEET
WALK

IRIS MAGNUS

THE
SWEET
WALK

Overcoming the

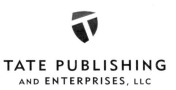

DIABETES
CHALLENGE

& Taking Control of Life

TATE PUBLISHING
AND ENTERPRISES, LLC

Published by Tate Publishing & Enterprises, LLC

127 E. Trade Center Terrace | Mustang, Oklahoma 73064 USA
1.888.361.9473 | www.tatepublishing.com

Tate Publishing is committed to excellence in the publishing industry. The company reflects the philosophy established by the founders, based on Psalm 68:11,

"The Lord gave the word and great was the company of those who published it."

Book design copyright © 2012 by Tate Publishing, LLC. All rights reserved.
Cover design by April Marciszewski
Interior design by Rtor Maghuyop

Published in the United States of America

ISBN: 978-1-62024-475-3
1. Health & Fitness / Diseases / Diabetes
2. Health & Fitness / Diseases / General
12.06.22

TABLE OF CONTENTS

Preface 7

The Summer of 1966 9

Diagnosis... 13

Clinitest Testing 17

Best Friend 19

Injection 23

Insulin.. 27

Diet 29

Disposable Syringe and Needle 33

Difficult Situations 35

Symptoms of Hypoglycemia and Hyperglycemia 39

Hospital Visits.. 41

Endocrinologist 47

Glucose Meter 49

Multiple Injections 53

A1C 55

Glucose Tablets 57

Vision Complications 59

My Love 63

Accident 67

Insulin Pump 71

Complications 77

Ketoacidosis 81

Glucagon 83

Why? 85

PREFACE

This booklet is written in hopes that it will be beneficial to those who have diabetes and their family and friends.

This author has lived with Type 1 diabetes twenty-four-seven for forty-five years. The booklet gives a brief description of the daily regimen with diabetes from 1966 until 2011. Also, how God has answered prayers and shows His care through the years.

There is a lot of information about diabetes and how diet and exercise will help us have good glucose control. Attempting to have good control hasn't been that easy. I felt it necessary to share my experience with diabetes in the hope it will help others who may become discouraged. A new diabetic and family may feel overwhelmed with diabetes. A person can live a good life in spite of diabetes. You will read about good times and difficult times that will make you laugh and cry.

At the present time, there isn't a cure for diabetes. It is my prayer and hope that we will soon have a cure.

THE SUMMER OF 1966

It was the summer of 1966. Our family lived a busy life in a small community of about 20,000 people. My husband was a police officer, and I worked as a nurse aide at the local hospital. I worked second shift, and my husband worked third shift. We planned our work schedules that way so one of us could be with the children at all times. Our daughter was seven years old, and our son was five. I was a twenty-seven-year-old female, weighing about 130 pounds and a height of five-foot-five inches. It was during this time I noticed I was thirsty as well as unusually hungry. My mouth and throat would feel so dry I got a drink of water every few minutes. When I was away from water for as little as twenty minutes I became extremely thirsty. One day when we traveled to my parents' about fifty miles away, I had not taken water with me for travel and early on this trip I felt I needed a drink quickly. I didn't understand why and thought to myself, *I am worse than my small children wanting to stop and get a drink all the time.* On the way, we passed an area where there was a spring running out of the hills, and I ask my husband to stop so I could get a drink. The water was clear, cold, and refreshing, but soon I was thirsty again. I thought, *This is really getting bad. I can't be away from water less than an hour without feeling I was going to choke.* During this time, I was losing weight and had gotten down to 120 pounds or less and looked unhealthy, with dark circles under my eyes. My friends kept telling me to stop losing weight. I didn't mind losing weight; in fact I was glad I had lost weight. It hadn't occurred to me to see the doctor. I had always been pretty healthy and didn't see the doctor very often. We didn't go to the doctor as frequently back then as we do now. I never thought of having diabetes and wasn't aware of symptoms of diabetes. Diabetes wasn't as prevalent then and very little information was available to the public. Some oral medications were available and a few types of insulin for treatment.

While at work one night, I mentioned to one of the nurses I was thirsty all the time and urinating a lot and very tired. So much that it was difficult to get my work done. The nurse asked if I had run a clinitest check. A clinitest shows if the patient is spilling sugar in the urine. I checked my urine, and I was spilling large amounts of sugar. I knew it was time to see the doctor. My advice to people is to learn the symptoms of diabetes and not put off seeing your doctor. A short time later, my doctor was on the floor making rounds, seeing his patients. While he was there, I shared my findings of high sugar levels in my urine. He set up an appointment for me the next morning at his office and ordered lab work. When I arrived at the doctor's office and checked in I was taken to lab to have blood drawn which was just a routine draw of my blood. The procedure was very much like it is today. I was sent back to the waiting room and waited until the doctor could see me. I had always taken everything pretty much in stride. Whatever the results I would face it head on and do what was necessary. Not knowing is sometimes the hardest to deal with. Since I already knew the results of the clinitest I knew there was a good chance I was diabetic. My thoughts went to one diabetic I had seen at the hospital who was on insulin injections and I had noted a combination of breakdown of her subcutaneous tissue of hallow areas and hard lumps where she had given her injections. I continued to wait in the waiting room and my thoughts went to more pleasant thoughts. Then I heard my name called to be seen. When I heard the results from the doctor I think I was numb.

DIAGNOSIS

It was confirmed that I had diabetes. After learning my diagnoses I was told I would need to take insulin injections. As the doctor and nurse gave me instruction on giving an injection and supplies I would need, I wanted to yell stop! Even though I had worked as an aide at the hospital at that time I knew very little about diabetes. I was feeling overwhelmed and needed a little time to let the information absorb. As I left the doctors office I felt like I was in a daze. After my drive home I began to feel better emotionally and thought, 'I can do this!' My glucose (blood sugar) level was extremely high, and the doctor put me on insulin immediately. It had been less than two months from the time I started having symptoms until I was diagnosed. The summer was hot, and I just thought that was why I was thirsty, and the excessive urination was because I drank so much. This is how I reasoned with myself until the symptoms went from bad to worse.

Keep in mind, this was the year1966. A person had to go to outpatient lab to have a glucose lab done. There was no way to check your blood glucose at home. I purchased a clinitest kit, insulin, insulin syringe, and needles at the pharmacy. No education classes were available. The nurse gave me instruction of how to give an injection. A small pamphlet was given to me to read on diabetes. Today there are many changes in diabetes care. Diabetic classes are available. These classes may last a week and education is given on diet, reading labels, exercise, what to do when you are ill, how stress affects diabetes and more. Other changes I have noted are glucose meters, many new oral medications, many more types of insulin, improved insulin supplies and insulin pumps are now available and improving. Today we have an epidemic of diabetes. One reason is because obesity is so prevalent in our society and many of those diabetics have Type 11 diabetes. Some diabetics with type 11 who loose weight by eating the proper diet and exercise control diabetes with oral medication and some control their diabetes with diet and exercise alone. Type 1 diabetes, also called juvenile or brittle diabetes, require insulin.

Diabetes is a condition where the pancreas cannot produce insulin or enough to break down sugar in the body. Insulin injections were given for Type I diabetes. Today, oral medication is available for some Type II diabetics. I have Type I diabetes. When I was diagnosed, Type I or Type II was unknown to me. I knew very little about diabetes. No one in my family had it. Not my parents, grandparents, siblings, or anyone I knew. I would search and read any information I could find about diabetes. I read the pamphlet that was given to me over and over. The information the nurse had told me about giving an injection ran over in my mind again and again. I wondered if I would remember everything. I read from our World Book Encyclopedia about history of diabetes and insulin. Computers were not available. I continued to feel very tired for a few weeks and then gradually felt better. My doctor had me return to lab frequently to check my glucose level during those first few weeks. This was done as an out patient. On one of those visits to the doctor, I picked up a magazine in the waiting room that had information about diabetes. I subscribed to that magazine which I received every two months. I was so thankful for more information about diabetes.

Today the best information I have found is through diabetes education classes. There are also booklets available that give us information on how many calories, carbs, sodium, and fats in foods we eat at home as well as many fast food meals and snacks. You can find these at some doctors' office, book stores and your dietician is a good source. Today we have a lot more information available through media, material and classes with other patients who are also learning about the disease.

CLINITEST TESTING

The clinitest is a urine sugar testing. It was the only way to check your sugar level at home. Following is a brief description of how to check if there is sugar spilling in the urine. A clinitest is checked by using a clean eyedropper and depositing five drops of urine in the test tube. Use a clean eyedropper and deposit 10 drops of water in the same test tube. Drop one clinitest tablet in the test tube, and it will start to boil. In fifteen seconds, shake tube gently and assess the color of liquid with the clinitest color chart. One could buy a clinitest kit with all items needed to run the test.

Sometimes I felt extremely tired, my skin cold and clammy. It was difficult to think clearly. Later I learned these were symptoms of low blood sugar and to drink orange juice to raise my blood glucose. When I had these symptoms, I would check my clinitest level, and it would show I was spilling lots of sugar in my urine. This was confusing because my symptoms were telling me my blood glucose was low. It wasn't until much later I discovered the clinitest wasn't accurate of what my body was doing at that moment. I would end up in the hospital with hypoglycemia (low blood sugar) or hyperglycemia (high blood sugar).

BEST FRIEND

It was a big concern when I learned a diabetic had a short life expectancy. The Lord was and is my best friend, and I asked him to please let me live long enough to raise my children. God answered my prayer with a big yes. The Lord has walked with me every day of my life, even those times I haven't been a good friend to Him. Prayer is simply talking and listening to God. One of my favorite songs is, 'My God and I' and it goes something like this. My God and I walk through the fields together, we walk and talk as good friends should and do; we clasp our hands, our voices ring with laughter.' This song takes me back when I was a child. I was a country kid and spent a lot of time outside. I loved to spend time in the pasture of prairie grass and lay in it looking up at the sky watching the white puffy clouds floating in the beautiful blue sky, and smelling the fresh prairie grass. Looking around I could see the wildflowers of tiny yellow, blue and white blooms. I felt the warm summer breeze. I could see and feel God all around me... My God and I walked and talked together. Our Lord speaks to us many ways, through His Word the bible, nature and people. My parents raised my brothers and I in a Christian home and were very supportive and gave us a strong foundation in Christian living. They showed me a strong faith in God. I accepted Jesus as my Lord and Savior as a young person and was baptized in the name of the Father and the Son and of the Holy Spirit. At that time I understood God the Father, God the Son but didn't fully understand what the Holy Spirit meant. Much later on a Sunday morning as I read the words, 'Holy Spirit,' I had a quickening within. Then I read John 14:16,17 NKJ. Jesus said, "And I will pray Father, and He will give you another Helper, that He may abide with you forever, "even the

Spirit of Truth, whom the world cannot receive, because it neither sees Him nor knows Him; but you know Him, for He dwells with you and will be in you." Having the Helper, the Holy Spirit who is my best friend along with a supportive family, church family and many friends has made my life a sweet walk. There have been some tough struggles in life but because of faith in our Lord and His love, mercy and grace we can persever.

My Helper helps in big and little ways in life.

INJECTION

The Helper was there when I was to give the injection. An insulin injection was to be given each morning. I collected all the items to give myself the first injection. I cleaned the area with a cotton ball soaked with alcohol, assembled the sterile glass syringe and needle, and drew up the amount of insulin the doctor had prescribed. Then I hesitated. Not realizing my husband was watching, I suddenly heard this deep voice say, "Do you want me to give the shot to you?"

I said, "No, I'll do it myself!" The thought went through my mind of when he gave an old cow a shot. When we worked cattle we often gave injections along with ear tagging, de-horning, doctoring and etc. When my husband gave a shot to the animal he would always thump at the injection site and then inject the medication. Of course he used a little more force because a cows hide is tougher than the human. I didn't want to take any chances of that force used on me. I could just see the syringe and all going through my leg.

After giving the injection, it was time to sterilize the glass syringe and needle. The needle was a much larger gauge than what we have today. I boiled the syringe and needle in hot water and then put them in alcohol and laid them out to dry. The next day, I would use the sterilized syringe and needle again and again, the next and the next, and so on. The needles would have to be replaced after a while, because they got so dull. It is a wonder diabetic's didn't have more infections from injections than they did. I never did get infection from injections in which I am thankful. A diabetic may get an infection rather easy because the immune system may not fight off infection. When the diabetic gets infection it causes their blood glucose to get totally out of control and usually they must be seen by their doctor and the patient will be put on an antibiotic medication to help fight the infection. If you have an open wound or injury the healing process needs the blood glucose in the proper range and with an infection it is difficult. Many diabetics have had to have their foot or leg amputated. They can develop a sore on the bottom of their foot or stub a toe and not feel pain because of numbness due to neuropathy. By the time the problem is noticed it may be too late and an amputation is necessary. A diabetic must check for any broken skin, keep it clean and watch it closely. Don't forget to check between your toes and the bottom of your feet. If you can't do it yourself, get someone to do it for you.

Before long, the subcutaneous tissue at the injection sites began to break down, even though I rotated the injection site. By rotating sites the insulin absorbs better which helps your diabetes control and there will be less chance of lumps or indentations at injection sites. Insulin is given subcutaneous, which is in the tissue not the muscle. The areas insulin can be given is in the anterior thigh, outer and upper arm, and abdomen, except not closer than two inches from the navel, and it can be given in the buttocks. Stay away from bony areas.

INSULIN

Insulin was first discovered in 1921. It was extracted from an animal pancreas. During the years, I have been on NPH U 40 beef and also pork, NPH U 80, Lente, and Regular insulin. Later years, insulin went to U 100. In 1982, the US came out with Humulin insulin. Humulin is biosynthetic insulin. It was thrilling when it finally became available. It was my hope of better control of my diabetes. Insulin is a hormone produced by the islets of langerhans of our pancreas and when it stops working properly or not at all we have a rise in our blood glucose and it can get extremely high, even causing death. Type 1 diabetics take insulin injections or wear an insulin pump to lower their blood glucose for the rest of their life or until we have a cure. Insulin pumps use a Rapid Acting insulin.

DIET

It takes work to control diabetes. There are many variables mentioned throughout the book that affects diabetes control for all diabetics and diet is a big part of diabetes control. At the time I was diagnosed the doctor put me on a lot of calories a day. I was put on 2000 calories a day which later was decreased. A certain amount of insulin was to be injected each day in order to try to keep the blood glucose at a normal level. As time went on insulin amounts had to be changed in an attempt to get the right balance of food and insulin to keep the blood glucose at the proper level. The doctor sent me to a dietician who gave me information on counting calories and eating a well balanced diet. She was great and very helpful. She introduced me to the food guide pyramid. Later, it was the food balance wheel. Both these methods help people with a well-balanced diet. I measured and weighed the food I was to eat. The way we measure and count the food we eat has changed for me. First, I counted calories. Later, the diabetic counted exchanges, then we used the point system, and now I count carbohydrates. The doctor will decide how he wants you to count your food intake. Remember a well balanced diet is important for everyone and the diabetic's food intake, medication and activity needs to balance out for good control. I say needs to balance and I am the first to say this is difficult at its best. Select a good doctor to guide you with your diabetes care.

My dietician and I started a local diabetic organization and had speakers come in to help educate diabetics on diabetes. The speakers gave useful information that was helpful to all those who attended. Support groups for diabetics are in several communities throughout the U.S. as well as diabetes magazines available with good information. Check with your doctor, the hospital in your area and/ or online when searching for a support group and information for diabetes.

DISPOSABLE SYRINGE AND NEEDLE

It really upset me that my subcutaneous tissue was breaking down at the injection sites. It upset me to the point I visited other doctors to get help. At one visit with a doctor, I asked him if he had any idea that might help the breaking down of my subcutaneous tissue. Suddenly, I started crying uncontrollably. It was a surprise to me when those tears erupted. The doctor suddenly had tears in his eyes and quickly left the room. I thought, *Now I've made the doctor cry*! After I composed myself and the doctor returned to the room, he asked, "Have you ever tried oral medication for diabetes?" I told him I hadn't. He said we could try an oral medication, but I would need to return the next day so they could run lab to check my glucose level. We did, and my blood glucose level was high on my return. I went back on insulin injections. Another doctor teased me and told me the areas I was concerned about were just dimples. As years past those areas of subcutaneous tissue breakdown filled in.

When I learned there were disposable syringes and needles available, it was a happy day. At first, there was one disposable syringe and several needles in a package. Later, they made the syringe with the needle attached. A new syringe and needle was used each day, and I no longer had to sterilize my syringe and needle. As the years went by, the needles were made of a smaller and finer gauge. The finer gauge needles were much kinder to the subcutaneous tissue.

DIFFICULT SITUATIONS

One evening, soon after I was diagnosed with diabetes, it was about time to put the children to bed, and I was feeling extremely tired. I told them we needed to lie down, and I would read to them. A short time later, I realized I was going to need help, confusion would come and go, I was having trouble thinking clearly so I tried to call my husband. He was on patrol. We had a CB radio in our house, and he had one in his patrol car. I called for him but couldn't say what I wanted to say. I later learned some friends who had a CB radio heard me making no sense. They called the police department and ask the dispatcher to radio my husband and tell him he needed to return home that there was a problem. I don't remember if I ever talked to him on the radio or when he came home. Later I learned my blood sugar was extremely low.

As time went by, I usually could recognize a low glucose symptom and treat it with orange juice. The symptoms with a low glucose levels varies. Usually one of the first symptoms I feel is being tired. My first thought is why am I so tired? After all, I had been feeling fine. Breaking out into a sweat is another symptom I sometimes experience. On occasion at night I will awake and unable to go back to sleep. I feel uneasy, and worrisome. I have learned I need to check my blood glucose at these times because many times my blood glucose is low. Changes in my vision also occur when my blood glucose is low. I might be reading or working on the computer and my vision gets dim. I check my blood sugar and usually my blood glucose is low. Anytime you have a low glucose treat it immediately. If you don't have your glucose meter with you and unable to check your glucose level, take some type of sugar immediately. It is better to treat the symptoms and have a little high glucose than go into a low sugar reaction and/or an insulin reaction. Still, the insulin reaction can sneak up on a diabetic. They can happen at any time, even after a meal. Many times after treating the low blood sugar, I had chills. It takes my glucose fifteen minutes to an hour to rise to the normal level. The chilling is worse at night. That is when my glucose level would get extremely low because of being asleep, and I was not aware of hypoglycemia. When I awoke, I was diaphoretic (perspiring profusely) and weak. I would treat the low blood glucose. When I gained enough strength, I changed my night clothes and bedding. Then I would have chills the next few hours. I find glucose tablets raise my blood glucose the fastest and that is what I normally use for an insulin reaction. It is better not to expect me to talk to you when my blood glucose is low. It will be difficult for me to talk and think clearly let alone explain anything. I get irritated easily when ask a lot of questions, I need a few minutes to recover after treating the low glucose level. With a low glucose level the brain is low on oxygen as well. The brain isn't getting the help it needs to function well. If I am in public it is embarrassing, and I certainly don't want anymore public attention than necessary. I have coped with diabetes and the difficulties like anything else in life, I do what needs to be done and move on.

SYMPTOMS OF HYPOGLYCEMIA AND HYPERGLYCEMIA

Hypoglycemia is a condition when the blood glucose is too low. Symptoms are listed below.

- Cold, clammy, moist skin

- Excessive sweating

- Dizziness

- Anxiety

- Headache

- Weak, fatigue

- Drowsy

- Difficulty to think clearly

Hyperglycemia is a condition when the blood glucose is too high. Symptoms are listed below.

- Extreme thirst

- Frequent urination

- Weight loss

- Constant fatigue

- Hunger

The symptoms vary, and a diabetic might have one or more of the symptoms at a given time. These are symptoms I have experienced.

HOSPITAL VISITS

We went to several different doctors, attempting to find ways of better diabetes control. A few times being in the hospital was something less than desirable. One occasion, I turned the call light on and told them I thought my blood sugar was getting low. The aide left the room, and much later, lab came in to draw blood. Later on, the nurse came in with a snack and said I needed to eat right away because my blood glucose was low. I thought, *Now you get in a hurry.*

Another time, when admitted to the hospital for uncontrolled diabetes, it was not a good experience. I called the nurse and told her I wasn't feeling well and thought my blood sugar was low. She said my lab had been drawn thirty minutes earlier and my blood glucose was fine. A short time later, my cousin came to visit. I remember her being there but don't remember much else. Later I learned she talked with the nurse and told her what she had observed, and then my cousin called my husband. It is my understanding that when my husband arrived he made it clear that I needed immediate care. He was told they had caused my sugar to drop on purpose. They checked my blood glucose. Yes, the blood glucose was extremely low. Some medical personnel had no idea how quickly a diabetic's blood glucose could change. We decided that in the future I should go to an endocrinologist who specialized in diabetes care.

One stormy winter night, my clinitest test showed I was spilling a lot of sugar. We contacted the doctor, and we were told to go to the emergency room. My blood glucose was high, and I was admitted to the hospital. The nurse stated they had several diabetics admitted that night. I said someday they are going to learn there is a connection with glucose levels and bad weather. Years later, I learned inflammation can cause the blood glucose to rise. Could it be when barometric pressure changes occur and causes inflammation in some diabetics? I have this question because many times before a winter storm comes in I have discomfort in my joints as well as a dramatic rise in my blood glucose. I don't have medical knowledge that the barometric changes affect the joints or diabetes but I do have that question.

One morning, when I got up to fix breakfast for the family, I was going to make biscuits and gravy. I was trying so hard to put ingredients together but had periods of no recollection. I remember feeling very tired. It was a difficult time. *Why?* I thought. I have done this for years. It was like my brain was in a fog of confusion. In all that confusion, I must have realized I needed orange juice because the first thing I remember that made sense was that I was at the table drinking orange juice. What a mess I had on the cabinet. It didn't look like biscuits. The family had cereal that morning. You guessed it. It was another severe insulin reaction. Over the years, I've had numerous insulin reactions. My insulin reaction symptoms have changed some over the years. I don't break out into a sweat as much as I used to. The tired feeling, vision worsening, and sometimes anxiety are symptoms I most recently experience. My husband used to say he could see a change in my eyes appearing less alert and a glassy like appearance. One time after the Timed Event at Guthrie, Oklahoma we were with our son and family and decided we would stop and eat on the way home. Before we got to the restaurant I began feeling like my blood glucose might be dropping. We got to the restaurant and I was pretty sure I was going into a reaction and I told the family I needed something with sugar. The waitress was busy but my son and husband got her attention and ask if she could bring orange juice right away that I was a diabetic with low blood sugar. She brought it quickly. In about twenty minutes I was feeling pretty normal again. My family is very much aware of how to take care of low glucose, but it is up to me to let them know if I have low glucose coming on. My husband has made the comment that he needs to write a book on 'How it is to live with a Diabetic!!' I now keep my glucose tablets with me. This is a good practice for any diabetic.

ENDOCRINOLOGIST

In the late 1970s, I found an endocrinologist specializing in diabetes whose practice was an hour from where I lived. It was then that I was put on two insulin injections a day and attended a week of diabetes education classes. Thank goodness for more education on diabetes. My husband attended as many as he could. It is good for the whole family to be involved in the learning process. Much of what we had learned up to that time was by trial and error.

The Endocrinologist is a doctor of the endocrine system. At your first visit to the doctor your medical history is taken, weight, vital signs, blood work up, urine check, physical exam including checking the feet. If you don't already have a blood glucose meter the doctor will want you to have one so you can take your blood glucose at home. The doctor will tell you how many times a day to take your blood sugar. Be sure to keep a good record of the time of day you take the blood sugar and what the reading is. This record will be good for your review as well as for the doctor to see on your return visit. Your doctor may give you a form to write your readings on. It will help the doctor make any changes in medication if necessary. Make notes of extra exercise you may have done, more stress, cold or virus, if you ate more at a certain time, or anything out of the ordinary. At your initial visit hopefully the doctor will set you up for diabetes education classes. More information on these classes was given earlier.

GLUCOSE METER

In 1982, I was working in a clinic and was intrigued with the glucose meter. It saved time to run a glucose test in the clinic rather than sending the patient to lab. I thought, *This is what I need at home.* My doctor and I visited about the possibilities of me getting a glucose meter. First, the price was so high it was impossible for me to get it. The doctor checked with my insurance company and convinced them the glucose meter was a priority in my life. The insurance company agreed and sent one to me, which saved the insurance company a lot of money and has been very beneficial to me. I haven't had to be admitted to the hospital for diabetes again.

The size of the glucose meter was approximately nine inches in height and six inches wide. It was wonderful to monitor my blood glucose at home. When I wasn't feeling well, I could check my blood glucose and know the glucose level and not have to guess what my blood glucose was. Like all other products for diabetes, the meter has improved. It only takes seconds to get a reading now, and the meters are so small they fit in the palm of your hand. It is impossible to express what a wonderful change the glucose meter has made in living with diabetes. Some glucose meter companies now give diabetics the glucose meter, which in turn you buy their glucose strips.

In earlier years, the autolet was not available, and one would stick their finger too lightly, not getting a drop of blood. Other times, they would stick the finger too hard. You then dropped a drop of blood on the end of the strip. The fingers got sore quickly.

To check the glucose level, wash your hands with soap and water, and dry hands thoroughly. Place the glucose strip in the glucose meter. Using an autolet with a lancet in it, stick your finger. Place the drop of blood against the glucose strip that is in the glucose meter, and the blood is drawn into the strip. The blood glucose reading comes up on the meter screen in seconds. I can't emphasize enough the importance that a diabetic have a glucose meter and use it regularly. Knowing your glucose and keeping your blood glucose in a good range to best of your ability can keep you from multiple complications.

MULTIPLE INJECTIONS

As time went by my insulin injections increased up to four times a day and I was mixing a long acting insulin and fast acting insulin for the injections. I had read about the insulin pumps. My endocrinologist didn't suggest an insulin pump and I didn't suggest it. The cost was tremendous and I wanted to see how well they were going to work before trying one.

The doctors said stress was a factor in uncontrolled diabetes. What are you stressed about? What am I stressed about? I had never thought of being stressed. Life in general can be stressful. How could I take anything out of my life that someone thought was stressful to me because of diabetes? I wasn't going to let diabetes control me. I will do the work I enjoy. A person needs to enjoy their work. Working at home, your job, driving, or any time there can be stress. People cope with it in various ways. I find I cope best by asking the Lord to help me through this period and I also have the need to keep busy. With diabetes I can become stressed when my blood glucose remains high or it bounces like a yoyo even though I am trying my best to keep it under control. I sometimes have to back away from checking my blood glucose so often. I may check it three times a day rather than seven times daily. If the problem continues I call my doctor for help.

A1C

Later, A1C blood glucose testing was done at the doctor's office. This test reflects your average blood glucose level for the past two or three months. The results will help the doctor make adjustments in your insulin regimen or diabetes oral medication if necessary. It also helps the patient make correction in his or her diet and activity. I was shocked how bad my A1C was. We made corrections, and I finally got it down from ten to nine then eight. Presently, my A1C is 7.4, with insulin pump therapy and I'm not satisfied with that level but I am getting there. The following is a brief description of Hemoglobin A1C levels for diabetics. At the present time the A1C percent levels are defined as follows:

- 6.5 and less is good control

- Less than 7.0 in people with other health problems like heart disease

- 7.0 and above is poor control

GLUCOSE TABLETS

Whether at home or at work, I would often have an insulin reaction in which there never has been any rhyme or reason of when it will occur. The hardest thing for me was to stop and rest a few minutes after taking something to raise my glucose level. When not at home, I used chocolate-covered nuts for some time because the sugar would work rather quickly, and the peanuts a protein/fat would kick in later. They didn't melt as easy as some candies. Glucose tablets are now available. I prefer glucose tablets because they raise the blood glucose faster. They are easy to carry in my pocket or purse. When the diabetic needs to take a glucose tablet, place the glucose tablet in your mouth, chew it just enough to break it up slightly, and hold it in the buccal (in the direction of the cheek). The glucose tablet will dissolve. It is believed that it works faster doing that rather than chewing and swallowing immediately

VISION COMPLICATIONS

One day while driving, I noticed the fence posts and signs looked crooked. This scared me. I called my vetreo retinal specialist's office and told them what I was experiencing. An appointment was made, and the doctor examined my eyes and said I had a bleed, and he would need to do a laser procedure on my eye. At this time, I had lived with diabetes about twenty years. This is one of the complications that diabetes can have. As the years progressed, I have had laser on both eyes, vetrectomy on both eyes, as well as cataracts removed from each eye.

My eye glasses have corrective lenses for each eye. The bifocals are set to read from my left eye. My left eye has the best vision. Large print books and my reading lamp with a natural daylight bulb have been great for reading. I found it difficult to read the numbers on my kitchen range. My daughter, who is an occupational therapist, suggested marking the cooking and oven controls with a marking puffed paint. A bright color of orange was used. The more contrast in colors, the better it is to see. The marking paint can be taken off easily if you desire.

My computer with the desktop widescreen monitor is helpful. I have increased the text size, which works better on a larger monitor. The larger monitor supports a larger resolution.

Driving is another issue one is faced with. I can drive in familiar places, but I am unable to read street signs until I reach an intersection. If I want to make a turn, it is too late to make that turn. When in unfamiliar areas, I no longer drive.

Sewing and playing the piano is something I always loved to do. Because of low vision, I am now unable to play the piano or sew very well. My daughter gave me an autoharp, which I love to play. I'm not an accomplished autoharp player, but it is a joy to cord by ear and sing. One must adapt to changes.

Low vision products are available. There are low vision businesses with many products that can help one to adapt.

MY LOVE

During the 1980's I took an Emergency Medical Technician course and worked part time for the ambulance service as well as working in medical clinics in Kansas and Oklahoma. In 1989, I told my husband I wanted to become an LPN, but I would have to have his approval, or I couldn't do it. He agreed, and I applied at two good nursing schools. I received a call from each of them to come in for an interview. I chose the one that was the closest drive from my home and was accepted. Here I was age fifty years old and going back to school. It was exciting to be accepted into the nursing program. I wanted to take care of patients in the hospital rather than pick them up out of the ditches. Talk about stress. I will admit it was stressful, and I studied hard. I didn't ace the nursing program but did come out with average grade of high B. About six weeks after I took the state board test for nursing, I received mail from the state board of nursing. I had been told the results would only say pass or fail. I was afraid to open it and asked my husband if he would. He did and said I had passed. He said, "I knew you would." We were very excited. I had already gotten a job, which was great. Nursing was my love.

Another love I had was to be outside helping my daddy and brother work cattle. My husband and I would help on some of our days off work. You just can't take the country out of a country gal or guy. One crisp morning, we saddled up our horses and rode to the pasture to bring the cattle in. The cattle decided to run to the south forty, and my horse Skeeter and I took after them. Suddenly, Skeeter started bucking. It took all my strength to try to keep her head up, which I didn't. I was leaning back in the saddle so I didn't go over her head. I heard my husband holler to head the cattle off. I thought how in the heck does he thinks I can do that on a bucking horse. I managed to stay on my horse and was not happy with the horse or my husband at that point. We got the cattle gathered and drove them to the gate. My dad was at the gate grinning and said, "I see you had a little trouble with your horse! I have heard all those words before but never quite in that order!"

Being active is important for everyone. I try to walk every day or do some type of activity to get the blood flowing. Enjoy what you do. When you have joy, you relax and it will help with diabetes control.

ACCIDENT

One day while working at the hospital, we got a call at the nurse's station that my dad was bringing my husband in. My husband had fallen from the roof of the barn and had a serious leg injury. He was transported by ambulance to a larger hospital where he had surgery. After surgery, the doctor said he had about 20 percent chance of saving the leg. I prayed and prayed he would save the leg. Many surgeries followed. He experienced a lot of pain, and a few years later they amputated the leg.

Eight months after my husband's accident, I was working late at the hospital. I looked up and saw my husband

and a police officer walking down the hall. I told another nurse that something was wrong. My husband motioned for me to come to him. We stepped in a vacant room. He then told me that my dad had been killed in a vehicle accident. There are not words to express the shock a person goes through at a time like this. The stress during this time affected the diabetes a great deal and my health in general.

A short time later, I began to have heart problems. I was admitted to the local hospital with chest pain. The nurse came in my room that evening and said my blood sugar was up to 300. She had an order to give me ten units regular insulin. I was about an hour-and-a-half from my diabetes specialist. I said my blood sugar would bottom out with that much regular insulin. She reported back to the doctor on-call. She came back and said she was told to give me the amount of insulin that I said. He told her that I knew my diabetes better than anyone. I had diabetes thirty years by then and had learned about how much insulin to inject to bring the blood sugar down. I told her to give me three units, and then we could re-check the blood sugar in a couple hours. I carried my glucose meter and glucose tablets with me all the time. The three units worked well that time. If there is anything I've learned about diabetes, it's that it is unpredictable.

The next day I was transported to a larger hospital and saw my cardiologist who found a blockage in my heart. A stent was inserted in the artery of the blockage area. This procedure is called angioplasty with stent, which increases blood flow. Emotional and physical stress affects diabetes. The stress can make the blood glucose either go up or down, to extremes from the normal range. Anytime any part of the body isn't able to function normally, such as the heart, it can affect diabetes. It adds stress on the body and anxiety plays a part. While in the hospital my glucose level raised to a high level then dropped. An endocrinologist was brought in who helped regulate the blood sugar.

INSULIN PUMP

In 1997, my doctor who specialized in diabetes suggested I start using an insulin pump for my diabetes. It was a good suggestion, but my insurance company refused to cover any part of the cost. I was looking at a cost out-of-pocket at around $5000 and then monthly expense for supplies. Could I really justify this cost? My husband and I discussed this and prayed about what I should do.

In January of 1998, I purchased my first insulin pump. A pump specialist from the company where I purchased the pump and the diabetes doctor gave me instructions to set up the pump.

The insulin pump is a small computer connected to your body that gives you insulin twenty-four hours a day via tubing from a syringe that is in the pump. It takes place of insulin shots. Rapid-acting insulin is used in the insulin pump. A needle is inserted under the skin in subcutaneous tissue. It has adhesive, to hold it in place, and you then pull the needle out, leaving the cannula in the subcutaneous tissue. The site is changed every three days.

My recent pump has three basal patterns that I use. I have set the pump with a standard pattern, which I normally use. Pattern A is used when I'm ill. Pattern A is set to infuse more insulin. When a diabetic is ill, they usually need more insulin. Each pattern is set with six different basal rates, which infuse throughout the twenty-four hours. Each individual has different insulin needs. You and your doctor work together on those needs.

At mealtime a bolus is given. The bolus on my pump is set with the bolus wizard and is set on a carb/ratio for each meal. I usually check my blood glucose seven times a day and always before a meal. The glucose reading transmits from the glucose meter to my pump. Before I eat, I count the carbohydrates that I will eat and program the carbohydrates in the pump. The amount of insulin to be given shows on the pump screen. I then press activate, and the pump delivers the insulin into my body. This is called the bolus delivery.

The doctor will make the decision of the amount of insulin to be given for basal rates, bolus amounts, on sick days, and various activities. The pump can be clipped to the waist band or a belt can be purchased and placed on the waist or leg. The pump has many features that I haven't mentioned here. More information about insulin pumps can be found on line. Since I have been using the insulin pump my A1C has improved. Like all other insulin products the pump continues to update. I like the pump because I only insert a needle every three days instead of three or four times a day. It is easier at meal time as all I have to do is press a few buttons rather than drawing up insulin and injecting. It helps a lot when eating out since you don't have to find a private place at a restaurant in order to take your insulin injection. The pump can be set with various basal rates that infuse more closely to the bodies normal insulin use. If you are considering an insulin pump think about the idea that you will be wearing this twenty-four hours a day, everyday. You take it off only when taking a bath or swimming. You will be required to take your blood glucose at least three times a day before meals. This is necessary in order to program in the amount of food you are going to eat, so the pump will infuse the correct amount of insulin. There are pros and cons to the insulin pump. You and your doctor will need to make this choice. It is my best choice. Above all I have better diabetes control with the pump. If you require the insulin pump it too will require a lot of education and the doctor will set you up with someone who can help you with that. Also, the company that you purchased the pump from should always have a twenty-four hour help line to help you. If a company doesn't provide that type of service don't purchase it from them. At various times the help line has been a big help to me. For instance, an alarm on the insulin pump stated I had missed my bolus. I hadn't missed it. I called the company and they helped me. My pump is set for a two hour slot around each meal, like 11:30 a.m. to 1:30 p.m. and I had taken the bolus at 11:28 a.m., two minutes before that time period started. Therefore the alarm system didn't show I had taken the insulin. The pump showed I had taken it in another location. Another feature the pump does is store all information when I take a bolus, how much and what time and etc. It stores all my blood glucose readings and the doctor can download all the information and print it out.

Questions are so important. Don't be afraid to ask questions.

COMPLICATIONS

You may ask: Why is it important to have your diabetes under control? There are many complications due to uncontrolled diabetes. Let's look at some of the complications. A brief description is listed beside the complication.

- Coronary Artery Disease–heart disease that can lead to a heart attack

- Retinopathy–diabetic retinal changes, hemorrhages of the eye and blindness

- Nephropathy-disease of the kidney

- Neuropathy–affects the nervous system, the diabetic can have decreased sensation of the feet and hands

- Myonecrosis–muscle damage

- Peripheral Vascular Disease–vessels away from the center as the legs and feet

- Carotid Artery Stenosis–narrowing of the carotid arteries

- Encephalopathy–disease of the brain

- Gastroparesis—a condition when the stomach takes too long to empty. It can cause the blood glucose to be too high or too low.

In November of 2003, while at work, I began to have chest pain. Several tests were run in the emergency room, and I was told they could find nothing wrong. The doctor on call said he didn't know what was wrong, but it wasn't my heart. I thought this was wonderful, but what had caused the chest pain? I told my husband on the way home that I just didn't feel right, but I did improve. On the weekend in early December, I had chest pain again. I felt rather foolish going to the emergency room again, since I had been sent home recently for the same thing. I knew if someone had told me of symptoms like this, I would tell them to go to the ER (emergency room) immediately. I went to ER and was in the emergency room a short time. I was told they would send me to a cardiologist by ambulance to a larger hospital about an hour away. After the heart cath was performed, the cardiologist said I would have to have open heart surgery. The next morning, I went to surgery. At this time, I had had diabetes for thirty-seven years, which could have been a contributing factor of the heart disease. I also have family history of heart disease.

Recovery went well. However, I wouldn't wish that surgery on anyone. This major surgery leaves you in a lot of pain and I will admit that I don't like pain. It felt like I had been run over with a Mac truck. I wasn't sent home on pain medication but my primary physician put me on pain medication for a short time. That got me through the rough time. Everyday I would gain more strength. Before long I was walking a mile a day.

KETOACIDOSIS

Diabetic ketoacidosis is serious complication. It is when the body produces very high levels of blood acid called ketones. You may see ketone bodies in the urine if you are hyperglycemic. Ketoacidosis develops when there is too little insulin in the body. Ketone strips can be purchased at the pharmacy, and the diabetic should keep them on-hand at all times. When the diabetic becomes ill with a cold, flu, or any type of infection, it can trigger ketoacidosis quickly, and the diabetic can become very ill. One must call their doctor at the first sign of ketoacidosis. A few times with a virus I have had ketoacidosis and felt very ill. I didn't want to eat, was weak, fever, and very drowsy. My ketoacidosis was high and I notified the doctor. She increased my insulin and I pushed fluids; I required more insulin while I was ill and as I improved I gradually decreased the amount of insulin that I took and the ketoacidosis cleared.

GLUCAGON

A glucagon injectable kit is a necessary item for the diabetic to keep available. It takes a prescription from your doctor. There have been times when the glucagon injection has been given to me. It is given when the blood glucose is low, and the diabetic is lethargic or unconscious. When my blood glucose is low, I choke easily. So beware if you or a loved one is hypoglycemic. Glucagon increases the blood glucose level. Usually, however, with the first sign of low blood glucose, I take glucose tablets. Diabetics don't always react the same when they become hypoglycemic. Hypoglycemia can sneak up on you very quickly. There are times when the blood glucose is 75 mg/dL (milligram per deciliter) that I might have symptoms of low glucose, and other times I may not have symptoms. Could it be how quickly the blood glucose is falling? At any rate, at the first sign of low glucose, I check my glucose level and treat it if necessary. Most times I recognize the symptoms of low glucose before it gets too low, but not always. Diabetes is unpredictable.

Some say the target for fasting blood glucose levels for the non-diabetic is 70 to 100 mg/dL at the present time. After meals, 130 to 140 mg/dL. For the diabetic the fasting blood glucose target is 120 mg/dL. A suggested value after meals is below 180 mg/dL.

WHY?

I have had doctors ask me what I ate to cause my blood glucose to be too high, and other times they ask if I had eaten because the blood glucose level was too low. One time, when I was a patient in the hospital with uncontrolled diabetes, my doctor came in my room and asked what I had eaten. I told him what was on my tray and what I had eaten. He then asked if I had eaten anything else. I said no. He said my blood glucose was high. I really wish controlling my diabetes was as simple as the food intake.

A family physician is important to have, and I sure appreciate them. I have worked with excellent physicians. However, if you have difficulty controlling your diabetes it is my recommendation to see an endocrinologist specializing in diabetes. Also, many general practitioners are not familiar with the insulin pump.

You may ask if I ever ate anything with sugar. Yes, I have and do. A medium-sized baked potatoe and a snicker candy bar has the same amount of carbs. The insulin will cover the potatoe and candy bar the same way. If I decide to have a milkshake, I make that my meal. I don't do this often, but on occasion I like to eat some foods individuals eat who do not have diabetes. Counting carbs has given the diabetic some leeway. Many foods have added sugar, like bread, cereals, and prepackaged foods to name a few. For instance canned fruits can be bought without added sugar. These fruits have natural sugar and the carbs must be counted. I read the labels and count the carbs on everything I buy. I don't make it a habit of eating too many carbs (carbohydrates) because I don't want to gain weight or use too much insulin. Some say insulin can cause weight gain. Or is it the carbohydrates you eat? Eating a healthy, well-balanced diet is important for our health.

It is interesting, I can eat toast, an egg, and drink four ounces of orange juice for breakfast and check my blood glucose two hours after I eat and have a good reading. The next day, when eating the same thing and the same amount of exercise, my post two-hour blood glucose can be too low. This type of thing happens again and again. The diabetic can only do the best they can.

Several years ago, one of my doctors thought I was having the somogyl effect. I will try to explain by using laymen terms. It is a condition when the blood sugar rebounds in response to a low blood sugar. The body responds by releasing glucose (sugar) from the liver. If this is happening the diabetic needs less insulin. One needs to discuss this with their doctor. It is possible I have experienced this however not all doctors agree on this. Many times my blood glucose will drop in the 40s mg./dL, and a few hours later it will be 300 to 400 mg./dL.

A key to living with diabetes is keeping positive and do the best you can do. Do not let diabetes control you. It may seem like diabetes is controlling you since you are testing several times a day, reading labels, and measuring food. These are helpful to living a healthy life so we can do the things in life we enjoy.

It has been a joy to be involved with the children and their activities through the years. What a blessing our children are. They are now grown, through school and college, married, and have children of their own. Now we have two great-grandchildren. I thank my husband and family for their support through the years.

Living forty-five years with diabetes isn't something to celebrate. I celebrate life in spite of diabetes.

To the diabetic, you may feel overwhelmed when you are diagnosed with diabetes and sometimes feel discouraged. Don't get down on yourself. If you fail just pick yourself up and do the best you can do. That is all we can do. Be positive, be healthy, enjoy what you do and do the best you can. To their family and friends, it is my hope this book has provided information that has been helpful for you to understanding diabetes a little better and the walk with diabetes.

This is The Sweet Walk of sugar diabetes and above all the Sweet Walk with the Helper, the Sweet Holy Spirit. My thanks goes to Him.